There Are Doctors in This House!

Julia A. Royston

Illustrated by Cameron T. Wilson

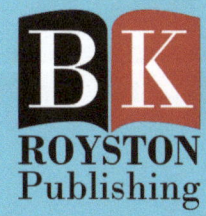

Royston Publishing

BK Royston Publishing LLC
Jeffersonville, IN
http://www.bkroystonpublishing.com
bkroystonpublishing@gmail.com

Copyright 2024

All Rights Reserved. No part of this book may be reproduced, stored in a retrieval system, or transmitted by any means without the written permission of the author.

Cover Design and Illustrations: Cameron T. Wilson

ISBN-13: 978-1-963136-64-7

Printed in the USA

Dedication

I dedicate this book to everyone in the Medical Field and especially current, aspiring and future Doctors.

Acknowledgements

I first acknowledge my divine and earthly teams that are with me every step of the way. I couldn't do any of this without you.

I acknowledge my husband, parents, family, friends and all who have inspired me to be my best in everything that I do.

To everyone that shall read, share, purchase and recommend this book to any child, adult and/or organization. Thank you!

There Are Doctors in This House

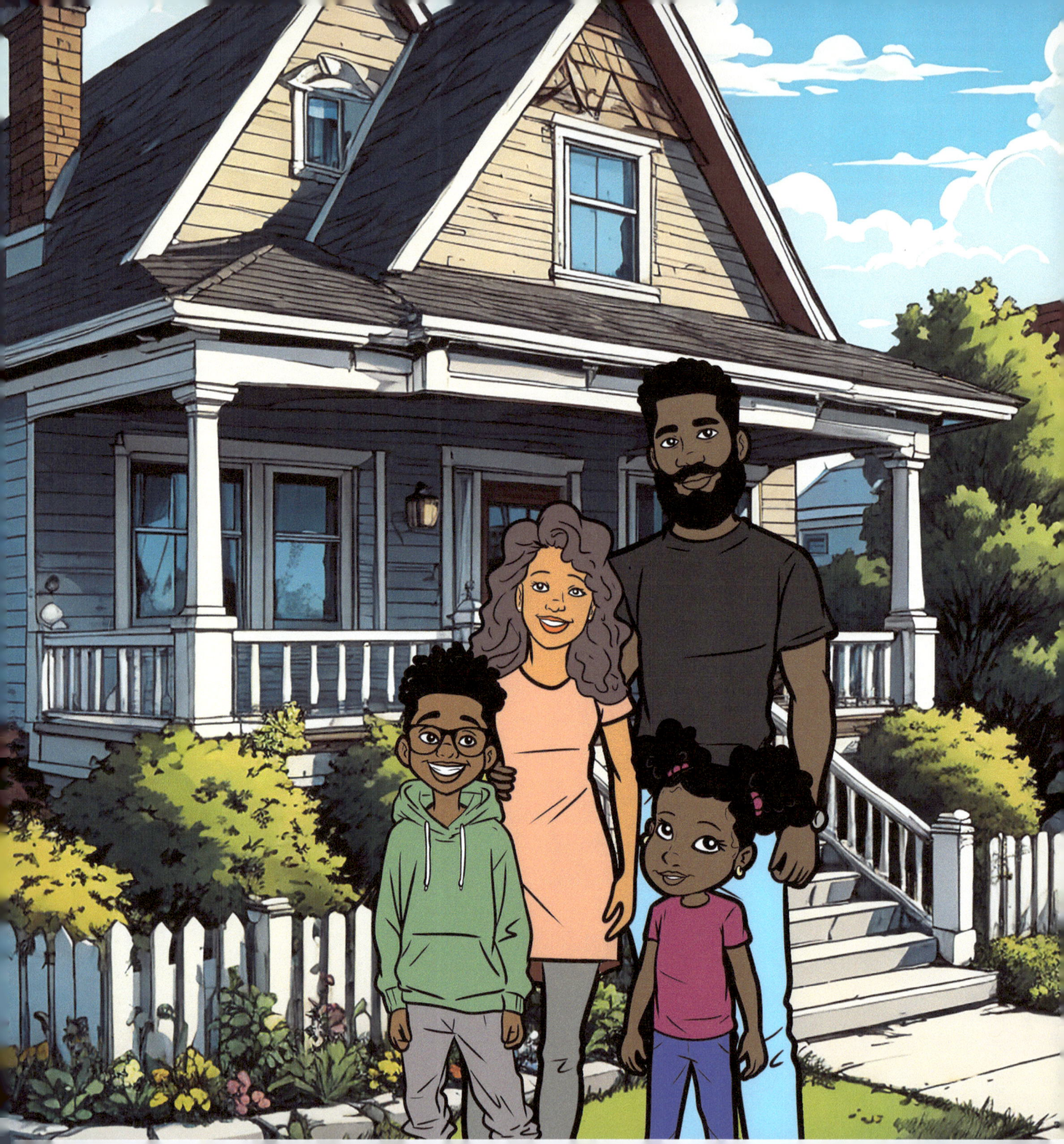

We're the Davis Family and in this House We're Doctors!

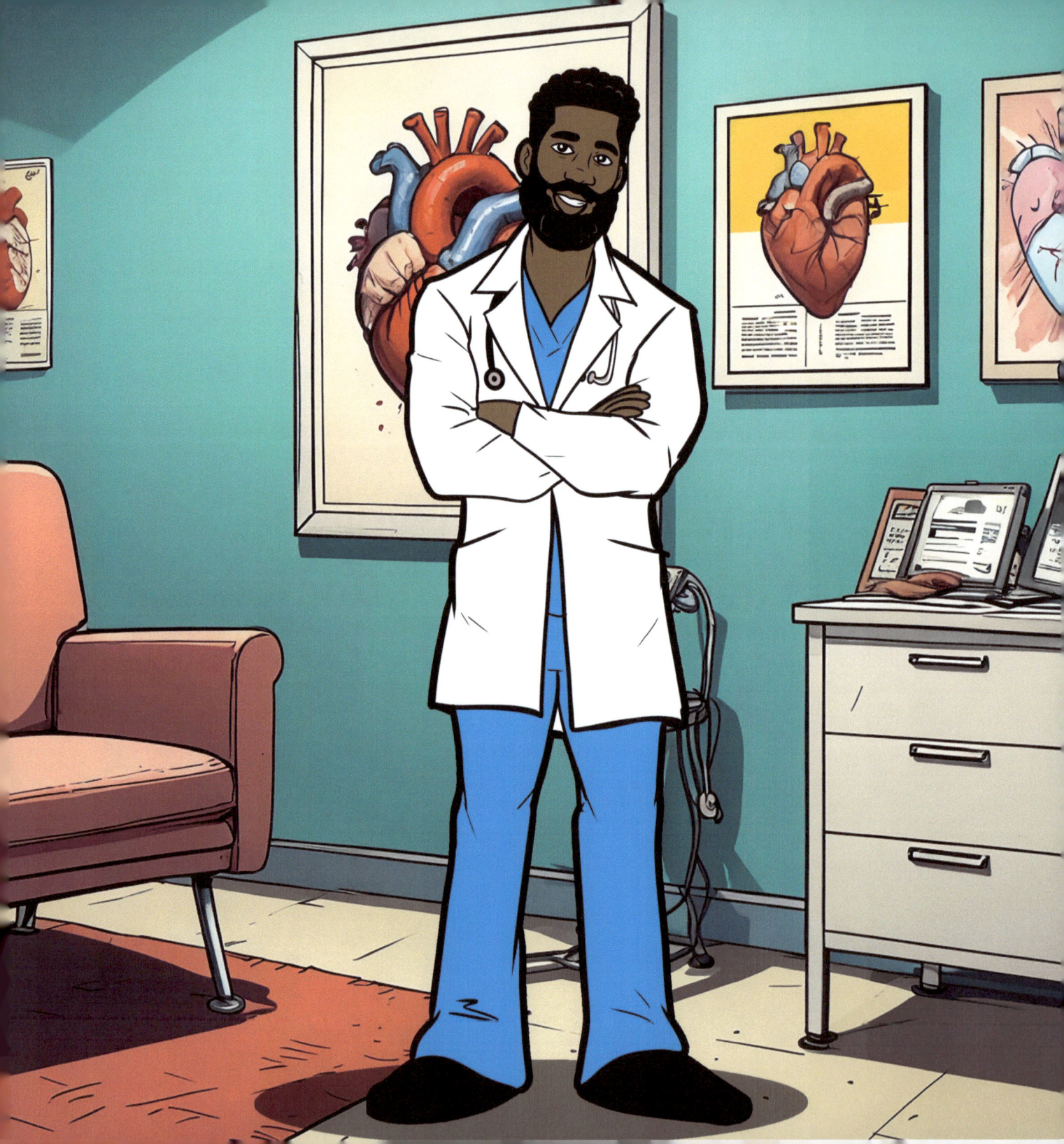

Daddy, David Davis is a Cardiologist!

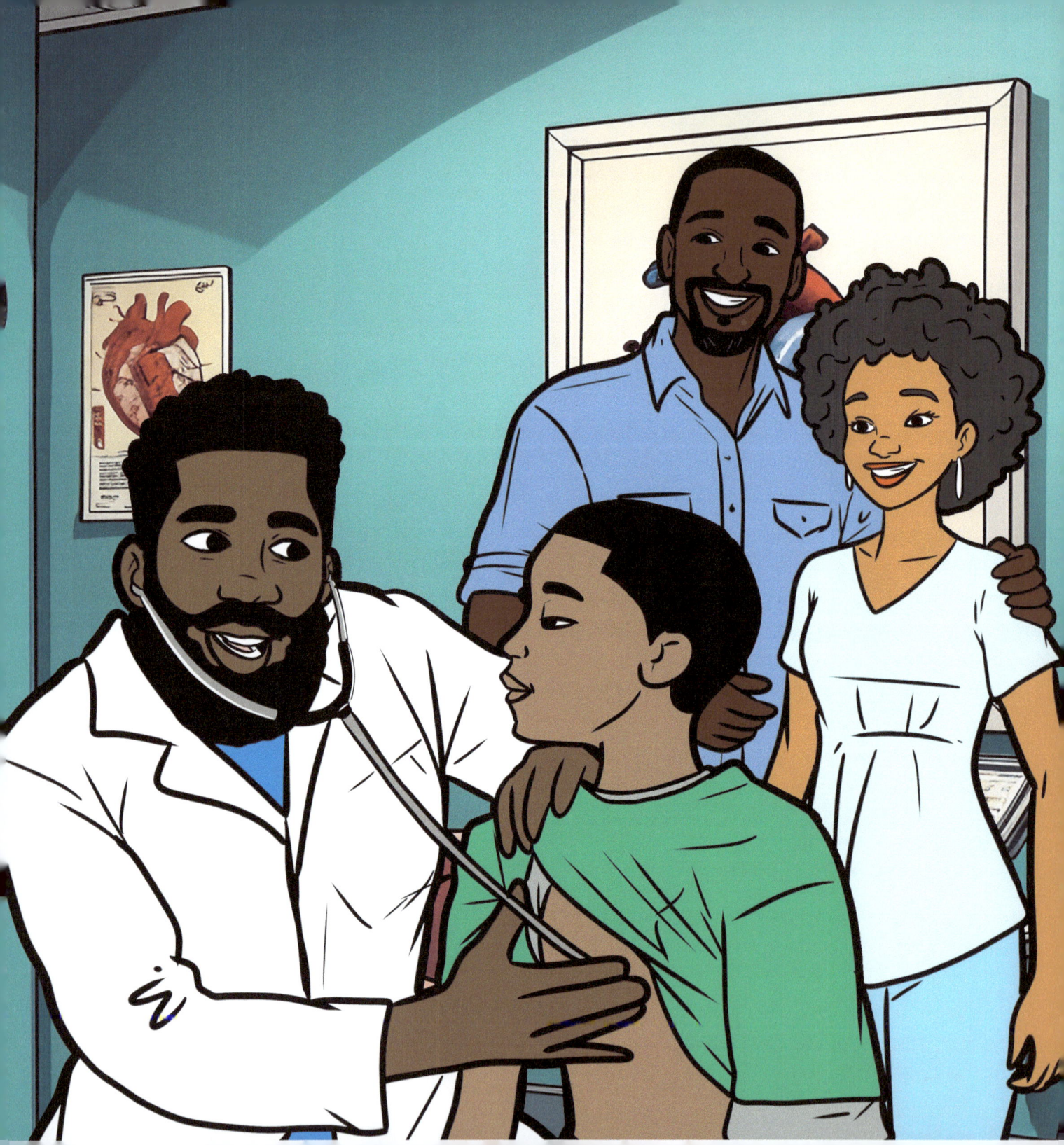

Daddy studies, specializes and cares for the heart.

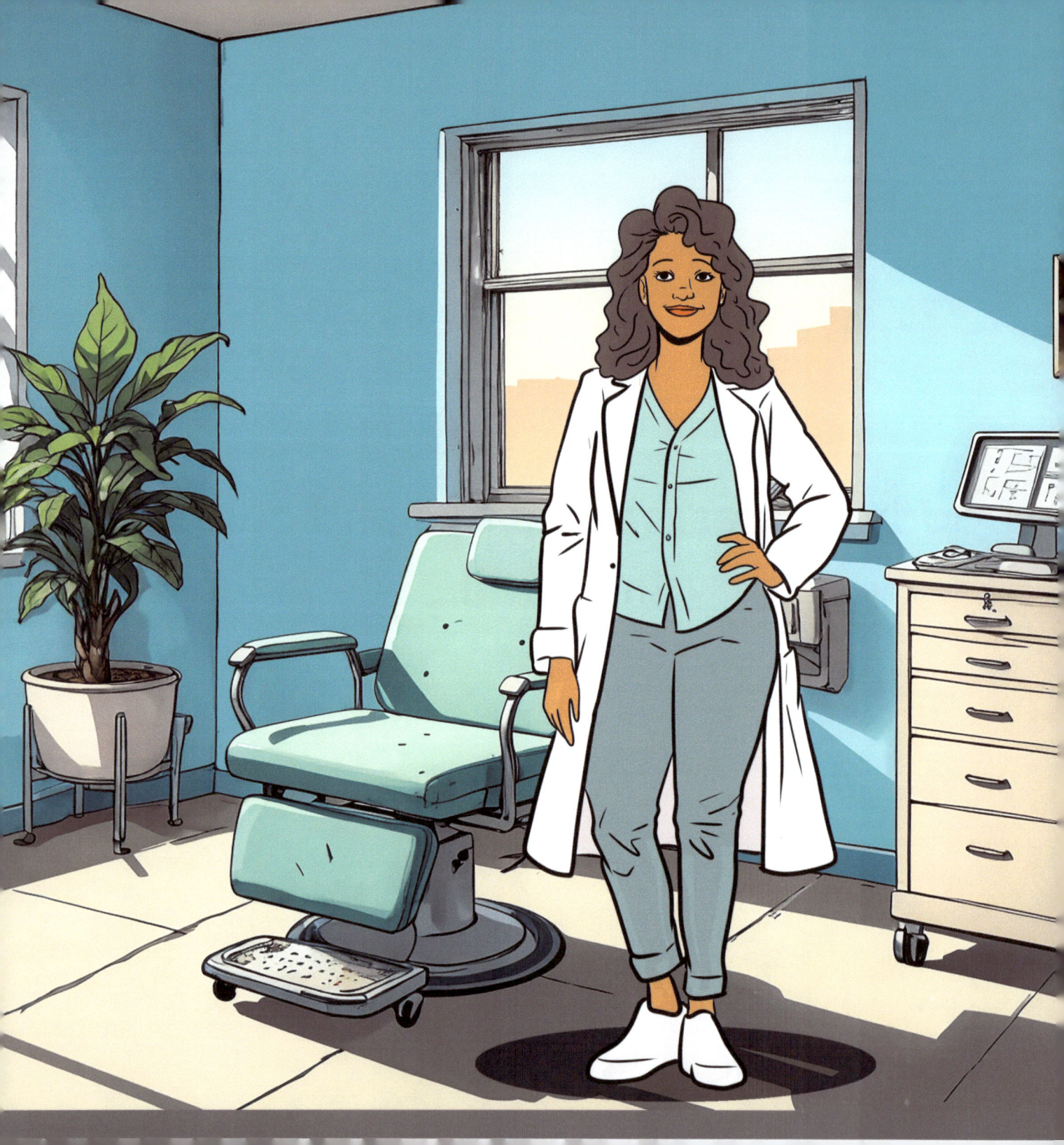

Mommy, Denise Davis is a Dermatologist!

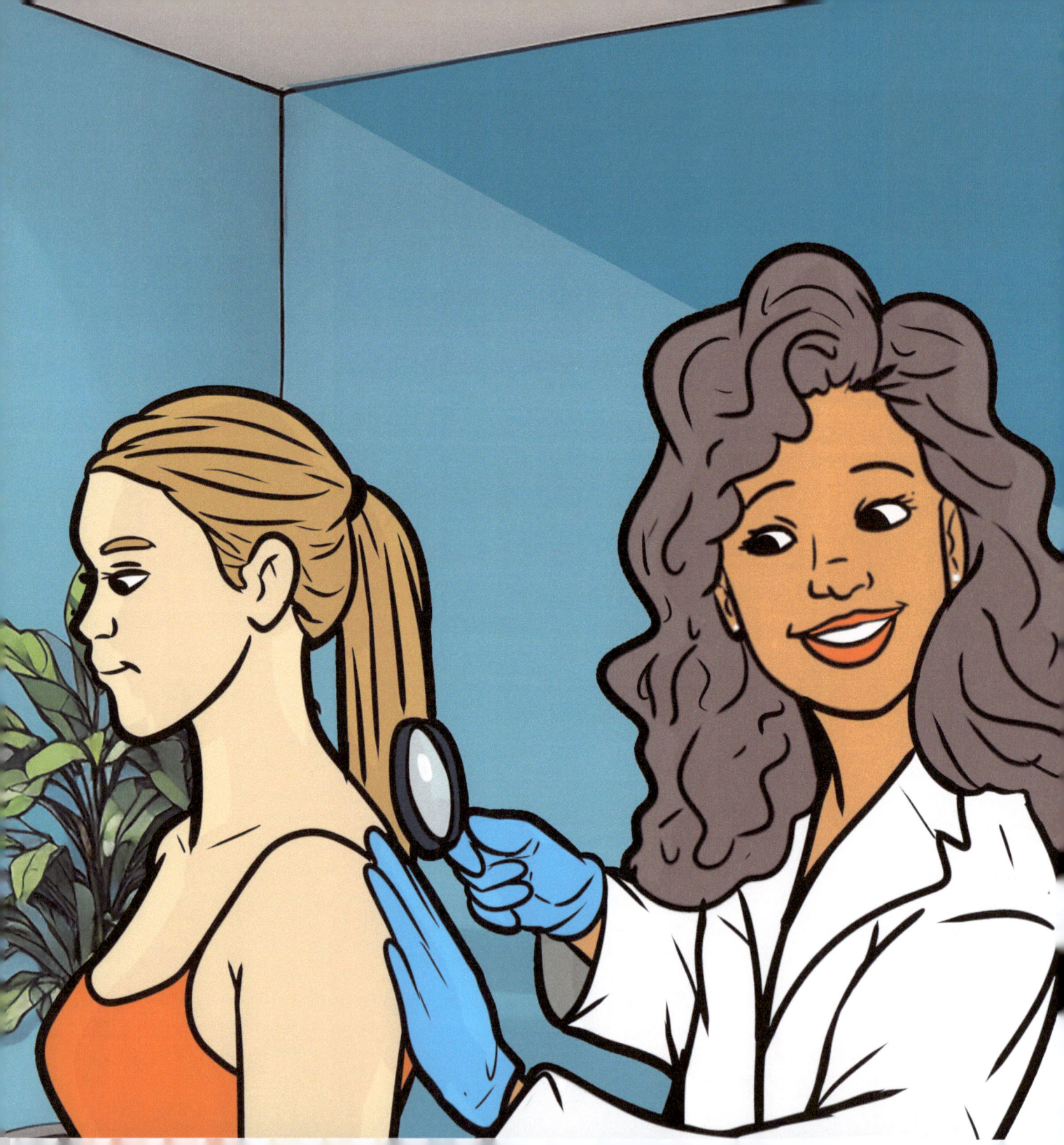

As a Dermatologist, Mommy cares for anything and everything about the skin.

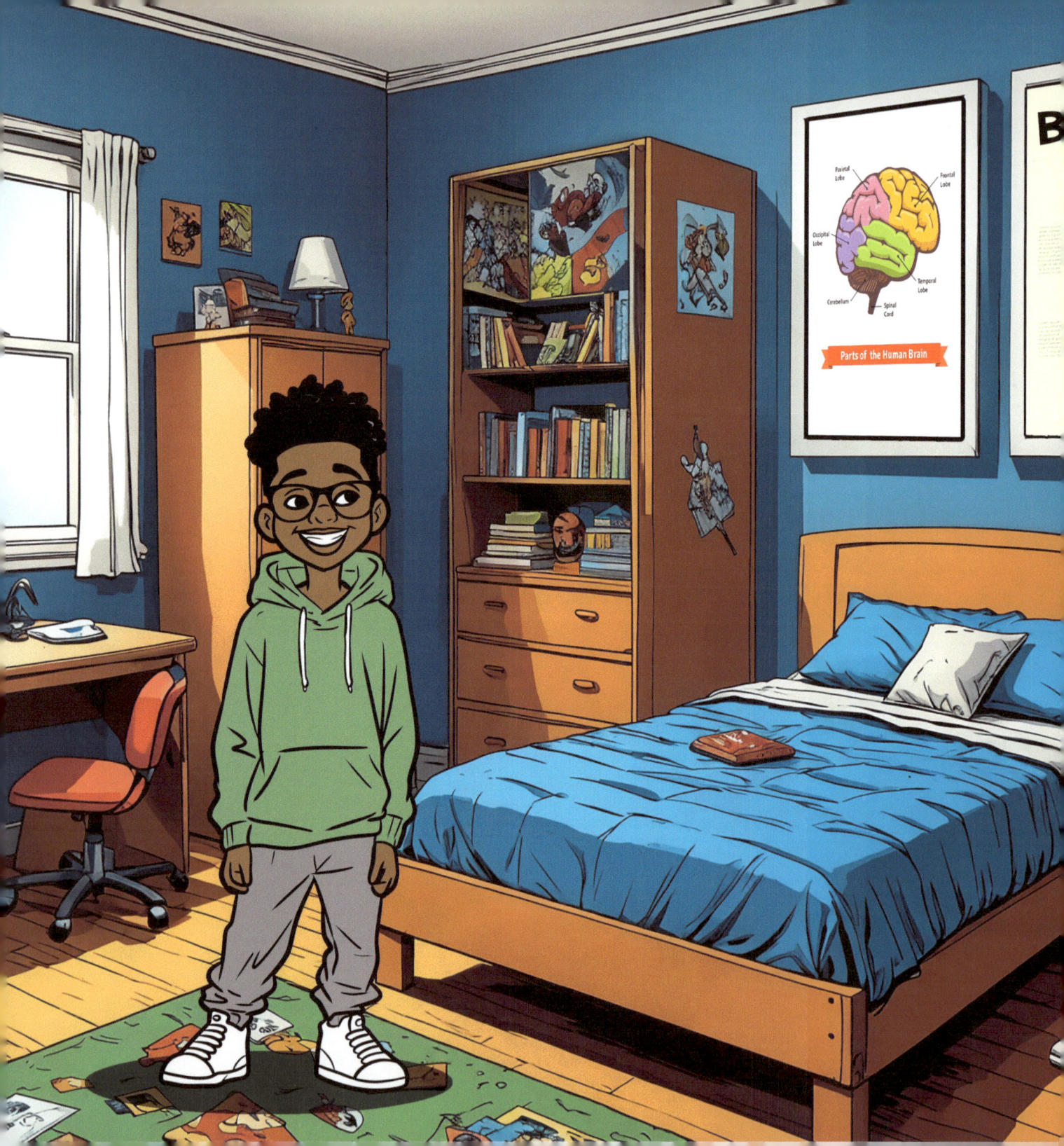

Dennis Davis will one day be a Neurologist.

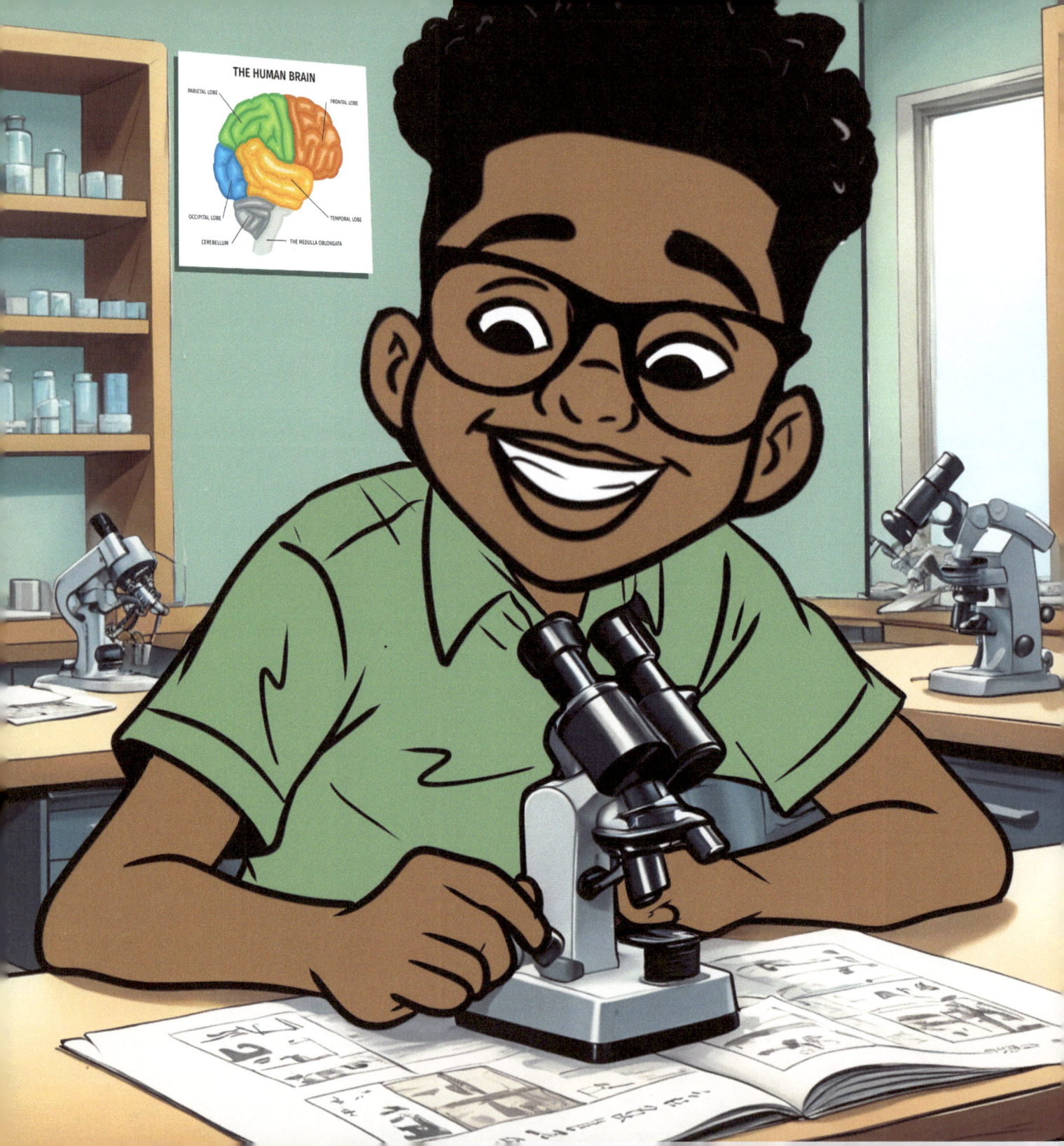

Dennis loves everything about science and the brain.

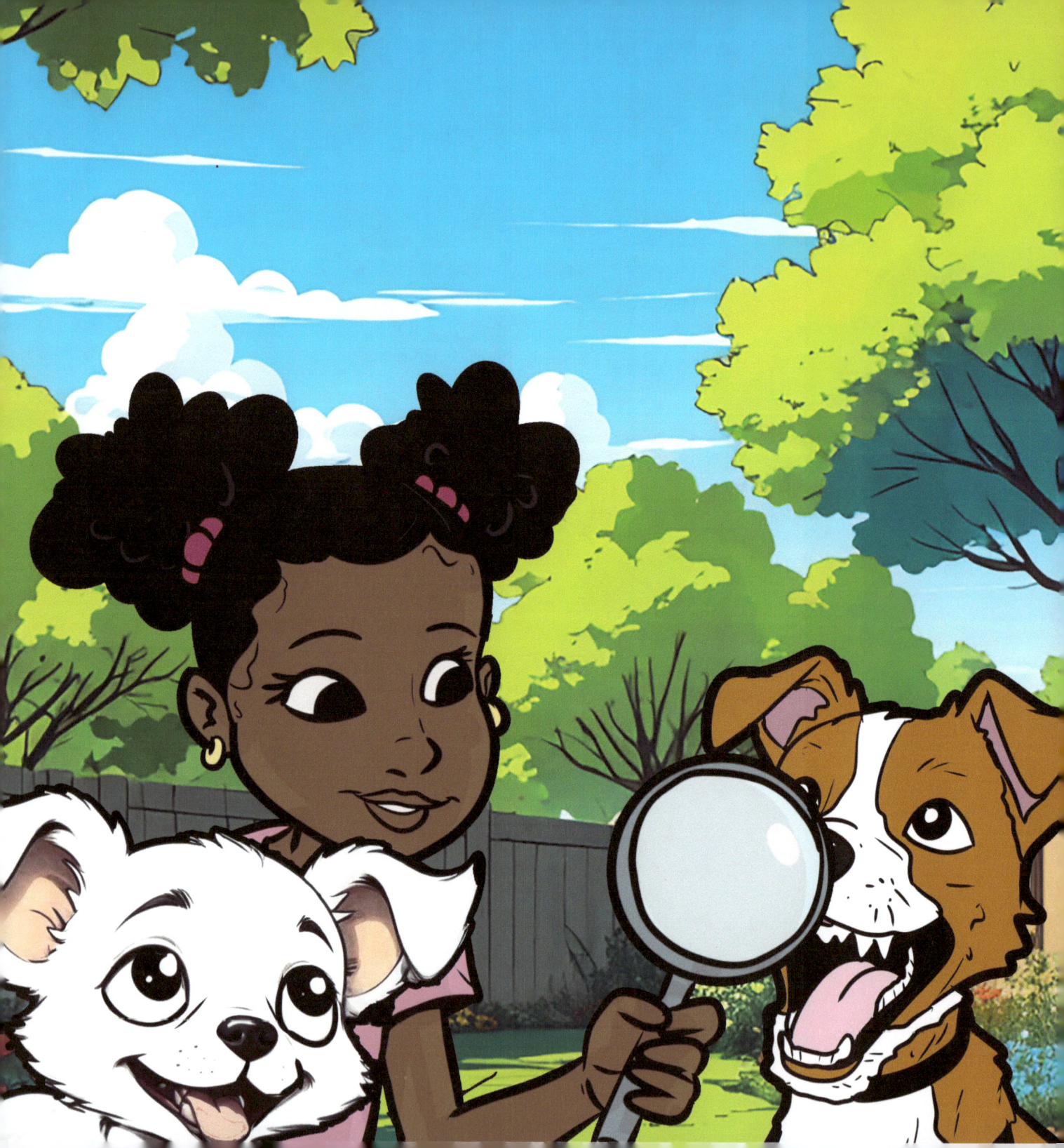

Devin Davis wants everyone in the world to have the best smile ever including our Dogs, Dynamite and Destiny.

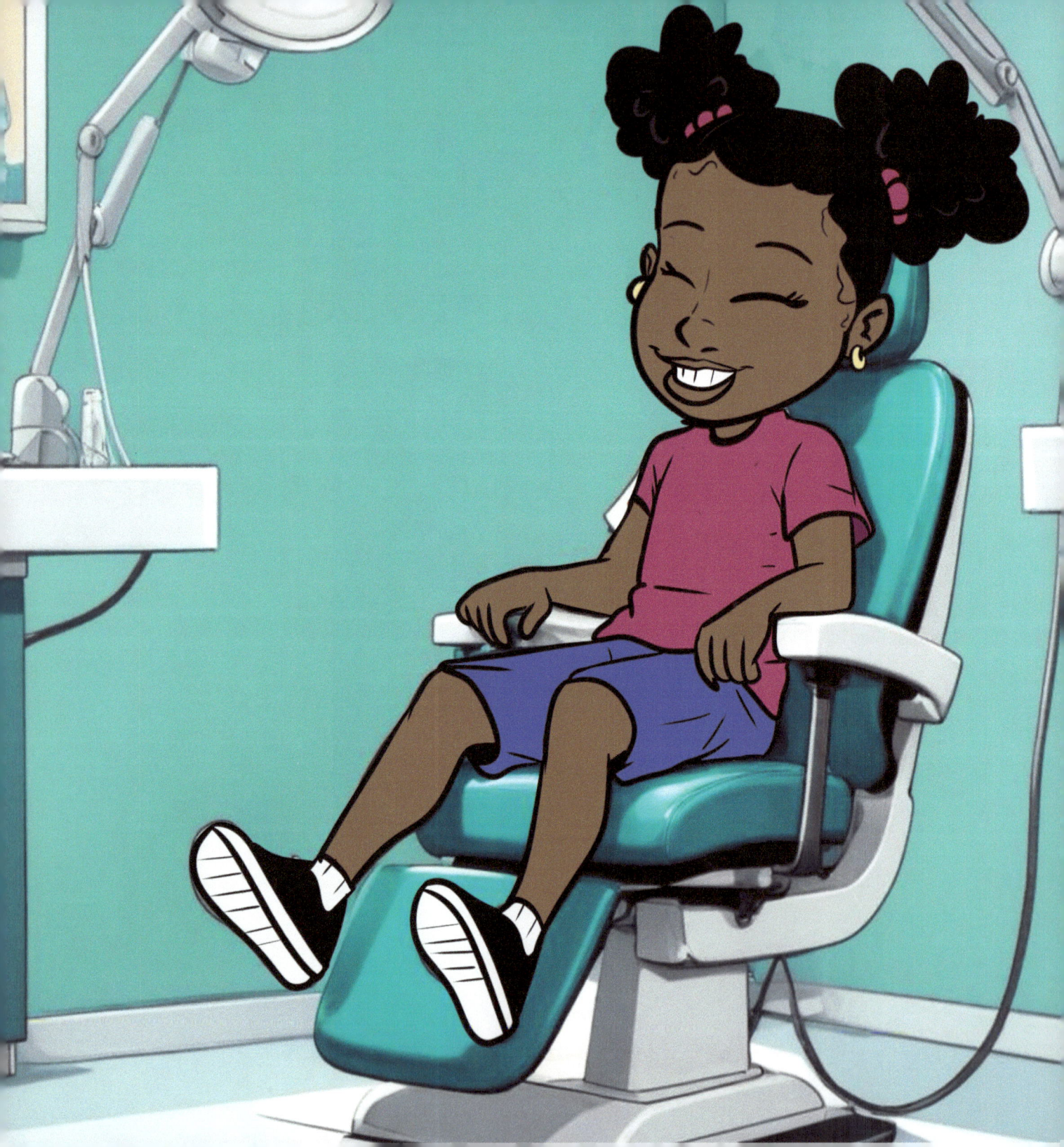

Devin will one day be a Dentist.

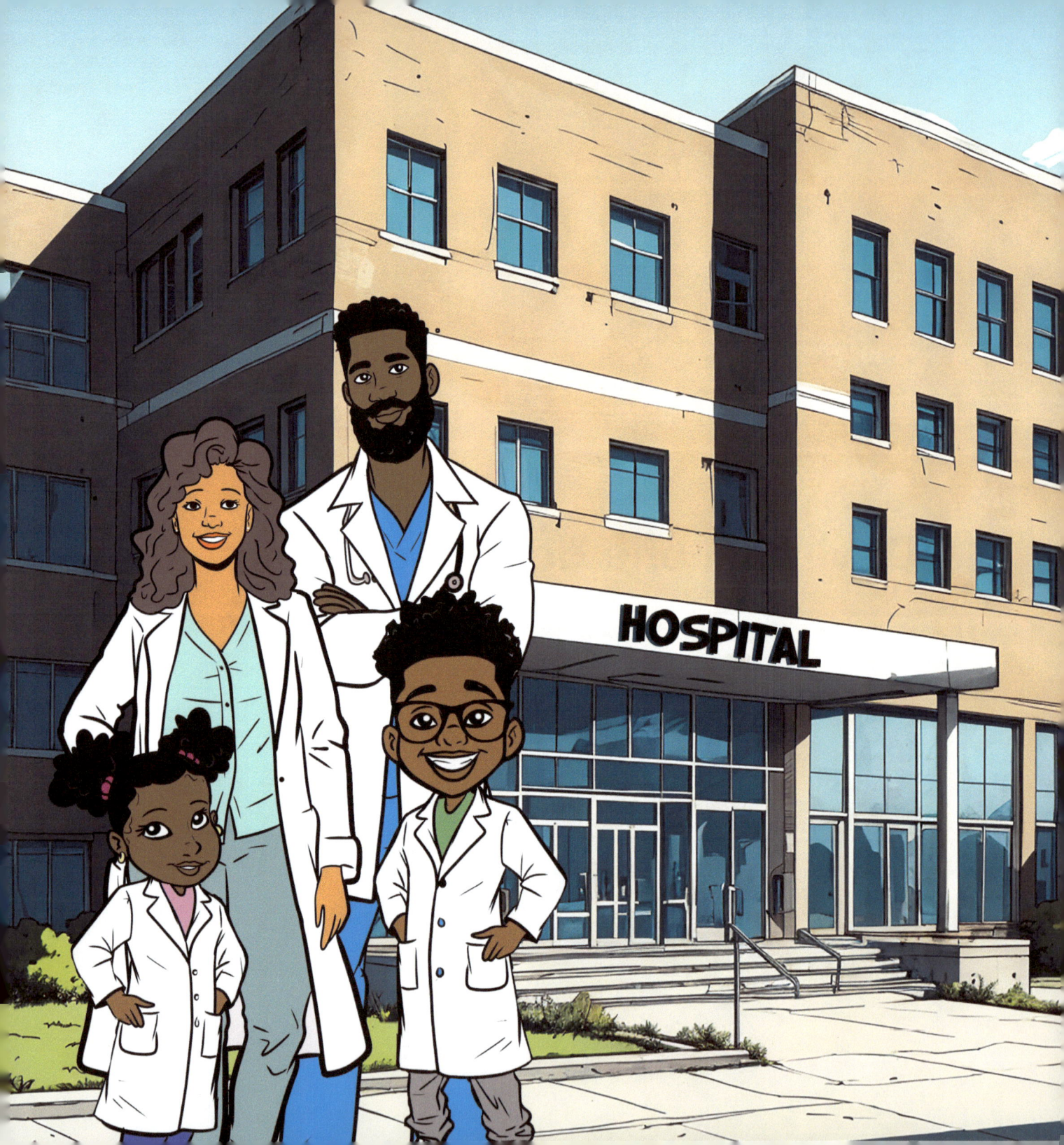

Doctors are very important in our lives. They study, research and help us to stay healthy, safe and strong.

The End

What do you want to be when you grow up?

About the Author

Julia Royston spends her days doing what she loves, writing, publishing, speaking about her why and motto, "Helping You Get Your Message to the Masses, Turn Your Words into Wealth and Be a Book Business Boss." Julia is the author of 120 books, published 400+, recorded 3 music CDs and coached many more to be published authors and business owners.

She is the owner of five companies, a non-profit organization and the editor of the Book Business Boss Magazine.

To stay connected with Julia, visit www.juliaakroyston.com.

Facebook - @juliaaroyston

IG - @juliaaroyston

LinkedIN - @juliaaroyston

TikTok - @juliaaroyston

Other Books by This Author

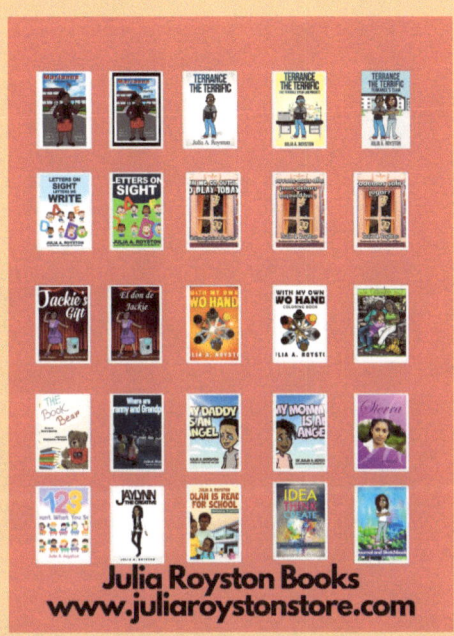
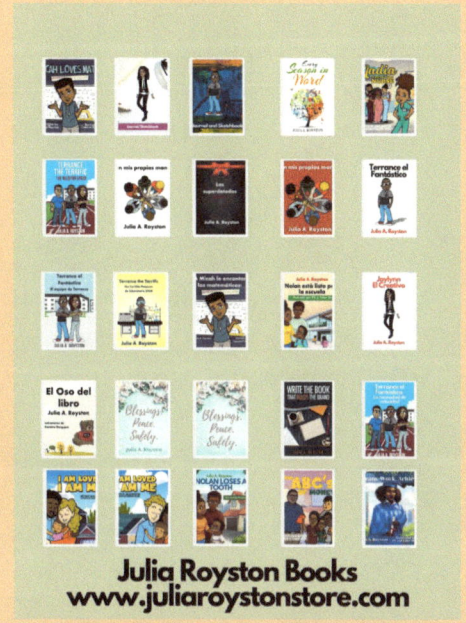
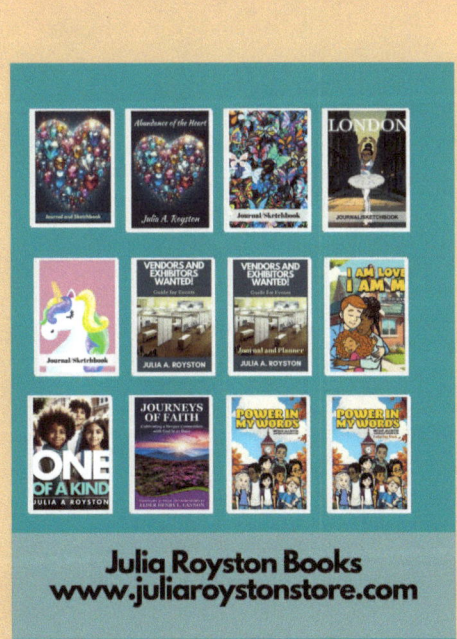
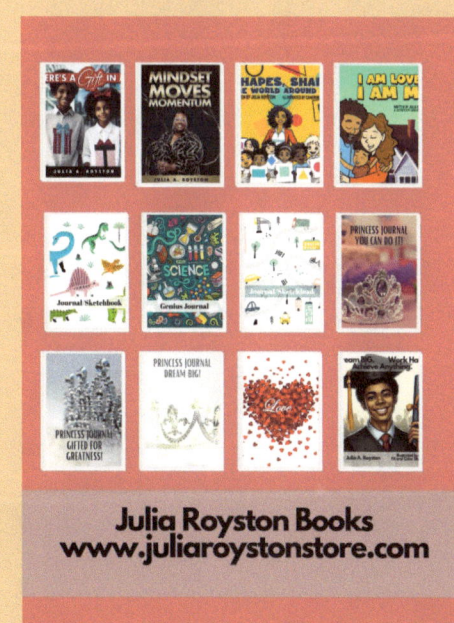

www.ingramcontent.com/pod-product-compliance
Lightning Source LLC
Chambersburg PA
CBHW061401090426
42743CB00002B/106